RECOVERY

RECOVERY

The Lost Art of Convalescence

GAVIN FRANCIS

PROFILE BOOKS

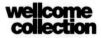

First published in Great Britain in 2022 by
Profile Books Ltd
29 Cloth Fair
London
ECIA 7JQ

www.profilebooks.com

Published in association with Wellcome Collection

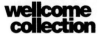

183 Euston Road
London NW1 2BE
www.wellcomecollection.org

1 3 5 7 9 10 8 6 4 2

Typeset in Dante by MacGuru Ltd
Printed and bound in Great Britain by
CPI Group (UK) Ltd, Croydon, CRO 4YY

A CIP catalogue record for this book is available from the British Library.

ISBN 978 1 80081 048 8
eISBN 978 1 78283 983 5

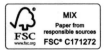

For my teachers
(in other words, my patients)

I enjoy convalescence. It is the part
that makes the illness worthwhile.

—G. B. Shaw

CONTENTS

NOTE TO THE READER

This is a book about illness and recovery, about healing and convalescence. I'm a general practitioner trained in a Western medical view of the body, and the reflections that follow are grounded in that tradition. Illness is as much about culture as it is about disease, and our ideas and expectations of the body profoundly influence the ways in which we fall ill. They also influence our paths towards recovery. A Faroese farmer, a Thai engineer, a Peruvian taxi-driver and a Sudanese schoolteacher will all have different traditions of the body and of health, and their paths to recovery can be comparably diverse.

What follows is a series of explorations of recovery and convalescence seen from within a particular medical tradition – my own as a European, twenty-first-century, general medical practitioner. While I acknowledge the value and the virtues of alternative approaches to the body and to illness, I will leave discussion of them to others trained in their use.

The patient stories that follow are either so commonly encountered as to risk no betrayal of confidence, or have been disguised beyond any possibility of recognition. Confidence means 'with faith' – we are all patients sooner or later; we all want faith that we'll be heard, and that our privacy will be respected.

1

THE LOST ART OF CONVALESCENCE

When I was twelve years old I had a stupid accident. I was cycling home from town with friends when a colossus of a lorry passed too close, causing me to swerve my bicycle. It was over in a moment: I put out my left foot to steady myself, and my heel jarred hard against the kerb. The impact tumbled me off the bike and onto the pavement where I lay in the dust, relieved to be alive, but unable to straighten my leg. The lorry didn't stop.

My pals pedalled off to get help, and after what seemed an age, but was probably only twenty minutes, my mum turned up to take me to hospital. An X-ray showed that the topmost piece of my shin bone, the 'tibial plateau', had splintered, and a fragment had become lodged at the back of my knee joint. And just as a sliver of wood can hold back a heavy door, that tiny fragment wedged my knee in a bent position.

I was taken to an operating theatre where, under anaesthetic, a surgeon wrenched the knee back and forth until that splinter of bone fell into place. A cylinder of plaster was rolled around the leg, I was given some crutches, and told to come back in the autumn.

To be immobilised in plaster through the summer holidays would have its challenges for any twelve-year-old, but it was once the plaster was removed that my journey of recovery really began. A metamorphosis had occurred. The knee had become bulbous, and my thigh and calf seemed by comparison stick-like, wasted and malnourished. A fine pelage of hair had sprouted under the protection of the plaster, bizarrely dark against skin that was now as white as bone. When I tried to walk, the knee wobbled and gave way.

It took months for my leg to feel like my own again; months of boring, punishing exercises to build up the muscle. Relearning to walk was a process led not by doctors, but by a pair of brisk and cheerful physiotherapists whose department I remember as one of too-bright lights, wipe-clean benches, weights, straps and gym bars on the walls. I can recall the distinctive disinfectant smell of the floor cleaner, and the regular company of a man I'd met previously on the ward who had shattered his leg in a motorbike crash. He was big, with a black moustache and stubble, and with a delicate gold hoop that hung from one of his earlobes. As we groaned and sweated together, lifting weights attached to our ankles, he joked about how I was recovering more quickly than him.

When I think of that period of convalescence now I remember afternoons at home reading in the sunshine, and doing my physiotherapy exercises at first tentatively, then with more confidence. The days were busy with sounds: of birds in the garden, cars in the distance, wind moving through the barley of the field behind the house. For twelve years my body had rarely stopped, and it seemed unnatural to have it rendered so motionless, as if with my injury the nature of time itself had warped and transformed. The flow of my life had been stilled, but it was that very stillness that gave me the opportunity to heal.

It wasn't my first experience of convalescence. A couple of years earlier I had woken one morning with a hammer-blow headache and a churning in my stomach. I suddenly knew the truth of the saying 'he couldn't lift his head off the pillow'. My GP was called for, a kindly man of the old school who took one look and, suspecting meningitis, sent me urgently to an infectious diseases hospital an hour's drive away, where the diagnosis was confirmed. I spent eight days and nights in that hospital, in a room with large windows that gave on to trees and afternoon sunshine.

In the niches of my memory I carry no images of the doctors, only one of a nurse in a sky-blue tunic, her black hair in a bun, her kind face lined with smiles. An iron-framed bedstead, glaring white sheets, and again, that smell of floor disinfectant. A window in an internal wall of the sick room gave on to a nurses' station – even when my parents were away I was kept under surveillance. Though my mum and dad took shifts to be with me for most of the day they also had my brother to attend to, and I spent many hours alone in silence waiting for them to come; waiting for home.

With a limb it seemed possible to objectify the part that needed recovery, to look down on the leg and say 'that's the problem, right there'. Working to build up the leg was effortful but also visual, my progress inscribed in the bulk of my thigh, the colour of my skin, the comparison with the healthy leg at its side. My recovery from meningitis was far more difficult to grasp, the edges of what recovery *meant* were far less clear. A languorous fuzzy-headed exhaustion dominated my days, burnishing the world with the bright haze of a dream or a hallucination. My body was in convalescence, but the process itself felt disembodied, ethereal, as much mental as physical. As I look back on it now, it's clear that it was my first experience of the complexities of convalescence, and how it can and must take very different forms with different illnesses, and between different people.

Six years after my leg recovered I went to medical school to train to be a doctor. A decade after that I was working in a brain injury unit, as a junior member of a team caring for a relentless flow of broken people – mostly young men who had been injured through reckless driving, falls or fights. I saw how quickly their bones could heal, but how much longer it took for their brains to do the same. Once the initial crisis of injury was over – blood clots removed, pressure relieved, skulls plated and wired – they would be moved to a 'rehab ward' where they might stay for months at a time, gradually relearning what were known as ADLs – 'activities of daily living': bathing, dressing, cooking and so on. For some, those 'ADLs' would include relearning to walk or to talk.

The word *rehabilitation* comes from the Latin *habilis*, 'to make fit', and carries the sense of restoration: 'to stand, make, or be firm again'. The aim of rehabilitation, then, was to make someone as fit as they can be, to be able to stand firmly on their own two feet. And though recovery was the clinicians' ultimate aim, it's curious that the words 'recovery' and 'convalescence' are generally absent from the index of medical textbooks. As long ago as the 1920s, in her essay 'On Being Ill', Virginia Woolf wrote that we lack a mode of writing about illness, that it is 'strange indeed that illness has not taken its place with love, battle, and jealousy among the prime themes of literature'. A century on, her assertion no longer holds true: we do have a literature of illness. But I'd argue that we still lack a literature of recovery.

The medicine I was trained in often assumes that once a crisis has passed, the body and mind find ways to heal themselves – there's almost nothing more to be said on the matter. But after nearly twenty years as a GP I've often found that the reverse is true: guidance and encouragement through the process of recovery can be indispensable. Odd as it seems, my patients often need to be granted permission to take the time to recover that they need. Illness is not simply a matter of biology, but one of psychology and sociology. We fall ill in ways that are profoundly influenced by our past experiences and expectations, and the same can be said of our paths to recovery. I have learned much from those other clinicians – the nurses, physiotherapists and occupational therapists – who have most helped my patients, and am always being reminded of how much there is still to learn.

The therapists in the brain injury unit knew that convalescence is anything but a passive process. Though its rhythms and its tempo are often slow and gentle, it's an *act*, and actions need us to be present, to engage, to give of ourselves. Whether it's our knees or skulls that need to heal from an injury, or lungs from a viral infection, or brains from a concussion or minds from a crisis of depression or anxiety,

I often remind my patients that it's worth giving adequate time, energy and respect to the process of healing. We need to take care over the environment in which we're attempting to heal, celebrating the importance of nature and the natural world and recognising the part it can play in hastening recovery. Many patients I've known over the years have found a way to make sense of even a very difficult illness journey. When an illness or disability is incurable it can still be possible to 'recover' in the sense of building towards a life of greater dignity and autonomy.

There is no hierarchy to suffering, and it's not possible to say of one group of conditions that they deserve sympathy while another group deserves to be dismissed. I've known patients whose lives have been dominated, for years, by the grief of a failed love affair, and others who have taken the most disabling injuries, pain, indignity and loss of independence in their stride. Though it can be tempting to resent someone whose illness appears to be less serious than our own, or to judge ourselves harshly when others seem to be coping with more challenging circumstances than we are, comparisons are rarely helpful. Neither should we be anxious to set out a timetable of recovery: it's more important to set achievable goals.

As a doctor, sometimes all I can do is reassure my patients that I believe improvement of *some kind* is possible. The recovery I'm reassuring them of might not be biological in nature, in terms of a resolution of their condition, but rather an improvement in their circumstances.

What follows is a series of reflections on recovery and convalescence gleaned from my own experience of illness, and of thirty years in training and in practising medicine. It contains much that I wish I'd known when I set out on my career, while acknowledging that there is always more to know. Every illness is unique, which means that all recoveries must also be in some sense unique, but I have tried to set out some principles and waypoints that have proven helpful over the years to guide me, and my patients, through the many landscapes of illness. It's a place that all of us must visit, sooner or later; from time to time we all need to learn the art of convalescence.

2

HOSPITALS AND RECOVERY

We need time to recover, but we also need a safe space in which to do it. A couple of hundred years ago there were few hospitals, and infectious disease was the main cause of illness. Convalescence, where there was time for it, happened at home. Throughout the nineteenth century it became ever more evident that offering a bed, and some basic hygiene measures, improved a convalescent's odds of survival. Between 1800 and 1914 the number of hospitals in the United States increased from just two to over five hundred. Between 1860 and 1980 the UK quadrupled its hospital beds. On both sides of the Atlantic these burgeoning hospitals were built on the principles extolled by Florence Nightingale, who wrote in her *Notes on Nursing* (1859) that hospitals should 'signify the proper use of fresh air, light, warmth, cleanliness, quiet, and the proper selection and administration of diet'. She also thought that the windows should look out on something green, growing and alive (a recommendation that has been borne out through modern research). She developed new ways of tabulating survival to better reveal the factors that most influenced recovery, and began to show that, when it comes to saving lives, good nursing is just as important as medical and surgical interventions.

In November 1854 Nightingale and her team of nurses had arrived at a military hospital in Turkey to find two thousand injured men dying in squalor – in those days more soldiers would die from infections than from bullets. One of her first acts was to order three hundred scrubbing brushes, and to requisition more nurses: 'I am a kind of General Dealer,' she wrote, 'in socks, shirts, knives and forks, wooden spoons, tin baths, tables and forms, cabbages and carrots, operating tables, towels and soap.' At the time of her arrival, one out of every two or three men were dying of their injuries, and although the military brass of her day disapproved of her efforts, they changed their minds when the death rate dropped to something more like one in fifty. *Convalescence* itself comes from a word meaning 'to grow in strength'. For Nightingale, this had an emphasis beyond the descriptive: the only way to beat infectious disease was to strengthen the body to fight it, keep wounds clean, and to optimise the environment around the patient to make it more conducive to healing.

Between 1879 and 1900 the bacteria responsible for the infectious miseries of mankind were identified at the rate of about one a year. As the biology of infectious disease began to be understood in ever-greater detail, death rates began to fall. And later, when antibiotics were discovered, the near-miraculous cures these medications effected meant that survival rates soared further. Slowly, through the latter half of the twentieth century, the idea of good nursing as the key to recovery began to fade. Time in hospital beds began to be seen as inefficient, wasteful and unnecessary. Some clinicians began to suspect that all that was needed was the right prescription.

Average lifespans around the world are now double what they were in 1900. But through the latter half of the twentieth century, as more and more of us began to live into years of frailty and dependency, hospital bed numbers tumbled. In the UK, we've halved the number available since 1988 (from 300,000 to 150,000), a statistic that's emblematic of a trend across the developed world. It's not possible for me now, as a GP, to admit a frail, elderly patient somewhere safe for nursing care and convalescence alone – the hospital gates don't open unless there's a medical diagnosis, and a plan in place that prioritises getting the patient out again as soon as possible. It's hard to get away from the conclusion that in the rush to modern medicine we've lost something important.

The same trend is visible in the care of mental health. The word 'asylum' once connoted a place of rest and of safety, but there are now so few mental health beds available that the 'asylum' aspect of psychiatric hospital is now available solely for patients so disturbed that their lives, or the lives of others, are at risk. Earlier in the twentieth century people were often institutionalised for scandalously trivial reasons, but the pendulum has swung too far the other way and it's now impossible for me as a physician to arrange admission to psychiatric hospital on humanitarian grounds, to ease someone's suffering. The only permissible grounds for hospital admission are those of safety.

If there is somewhere safe, clean and warm to recover, no one would choose hospital over home. But the recent (and at the time of writing, ongoing) pandemic has revealed cracks in the structure of medicine, health and care, and brought many long-term problems into a short-term focus. We have the opportunity as a society to do more than simply paper over those cracks: to finally rediscover the importance of giving adequate time *and* space to convalescence.

3

SNAKES AND LADDERS

You might not find 'convalescence' or 'recovery' as a heading in the medical textbooks, but you will find 'post-viral fatigue'. The association of infectious illness with tiredness was well known to physicians as far back as the days of the ancient Greeks: the first medical writings are full of accounts of fever accompanied by debilitating fatigue. In my medical work I sometimes see viral infections sending their sufferers to bed for weeks or months, and, in a few cases, for years. Why this happens is poorly understood: it's as if the struggle with illness draws so deeply on one's inner reserves of strength that the body does all it can to retain its energies, even going so far as to manipulate our sense of effort so that to take a short walk, or to climb a flight of stairs, is to risk exhaustion. In the periods of recovery from waves of Covid-19 throughout 2020 and 2021 I spoke to many patients in whom coronavirus had triggered this kind of enduring fatigue.

But if we don't push at the limits of what we can do in terms of physical effort, the realm of the possible begins to shrink, horizons contract, our muscles weaken, and sufferers can become trapped in a cycle of effort followed by collapse. The effort required to provoke each collapse begins to dwindle. Physiotherapists of rehabilitation call this 'the boom–bust cycle', and I've always pictured it as a kind of bodily 'snakes and ladders'.

Snakes and ladders is an ancient Indian board game in which the player makes slow progress up the board by making throws of dice. To land on a 'ladder' means getting a boost towards the top, but to land on a 'snake' means slipping back down towards the bottom. It seems as good a metaphor for the roller coaster of recovery as any.

But in truth life is not a game, and recovery is not snakes and ladders, not least because, in the game, all we have to guide our progress are throws of the dice. But in life, each journey up and down the board is propelled in part by our choices, not chance, and each journey up and down the board offers valuable experience. With each slide back into illness, we learn new strategies and become aware of new triggers that will help guide us, with more wisdom, next time.

Recovery and comparisons don't mix: everyone has a different tempo of convalescence and will require different strategies. It's *normal* that the process can be slow, and normal too for long-term illness to manifest differently in different people. Long-term symptoms from viral infections will be different for everyone, but can include varying amounts of breathlessness, difficulty concentrating, forgetfulness, mood changes, insomnia, weight loss, exhaustion, muscle weakness, joint stiffness and flashbacks.

All these are to be considered normal – not evidence that recovery has stalled or is going into reverse. On the contrary, those symptoms are evidence that the body and mind are reacting and changing in response to the illness. And where there's change there's hope.

The Greek physician Galen was doctor to the gladiators, and, as you'd expect from someone charged with patching up those who'd survived tiger maulings, sword wounds, and being clubbed on the head, he was particularly preoccupied with ideas of recovery. One of his books details the ways in which exercise has to be built up slowly after injury. Ball games, he wrote, are excellent training, because they use every part of the body and can be practised by all ages, the weak and the strong. He acknowledged that physicians of his time were often puzzled about which exercises were best for recovering strength in convalescence – puzzlement that I've found often among my patients today, who have to be reassured that it's acceptable to listen to their own feelings of strength and fatigue, of vigour and relative effort. Convalescence insists that we acquire a new language of the body, and I encourage people to learn its vocabulary.

The booklet I hand out to patients who are recovering from prolonged symptoms following Covid pneumonia emphasises the importance of this 'pacing', which is described as the opposite of the 'boom and bust' approach. It is 'learning to recognise how much you can do so you avoid feeling exhausted'. Someone in recovery needs to learn to listen to their own body so that they can begin to slow down and stop an activity *before* they begin to exhaust their energies. Stopping in time means that they will probably be able to begin it again more quickly after a rest. 'Pacing is especially important when you are breathless or tired,' it says.

The key features the physiotherapists of recovery would want the convalescent to adopt are relevant for anyone recuperating from serious illness, and are worth spelling out:

- Plan rests regularly throughout the day.
- Don't rush.
- Keep meals small.

- Don't plan anything within an hour of eating.
- If you're breathless, learn to control your breathing (physiotherapists will teach you these techniques).
- Get fresh air.
- Sit down often (even during washing, dressing, cooking, with chairs or stools placed strategically around the house).
- Drying yourself can be exhausting – use a bathrobe.
- Use aids to avoid bending and reaching.
- Push don't pull, slide don't lift, and if you must lift something, do it with your knees bent and your back straight.
- Don't do more than one thing at a time.
- Set achievable goals, little and often, every day.

4

PERMISSION TO RECOVER

When I started out as a GP in Edinburgh there was a story told about one of my predecessors. The story came from thirty or forty years ago, the era of single-handed practices, and the GP was overworked. To reduce the pressure on his appointments he devised a method of dealing with sick-note certificate requests: every week he'd pre-sign one pile of blanks granting a week off work, and another pile granting four weeks off. Then he'd go out on his rounds, and leave the receptionists to distribute the notes as they saw fit. This approach, I heard, had a happy side effect: patients who had previously been rude or aggressive towards the reception-ists became polite and respectful overnight.

Sickness certificates are something GPs have almost no training in providing, and are, in essence, prescriptions to take time off work to rest. Doctors are in a contradictory position: obliged by law to provide the government with judgements about capacity to work, but also obliged by their professional regulator to 'work in partnership with patients' and 'make the care of your patient your first concern'. We are supposed to work hard to maintain our therapeutic relationship with our patients, an ambition that can sometimes be at odds with the state's request that we pass judgement over them. Adrian Massey, an occupational health doctor who has written about this inherent paradox in doctors' roles, sums up the situation as 'doctors make terrible referees, but excellent coaches'.

In 2013 a social attitudes survey found that over 80 per cent of people agreed with the statement 'a large number of people these days falsely claim benefits'. But the UK government says that just 1.7 per cent of sickness benefit claims are fraudulent. Of those 1.7 per cent, a full third are thought to be over-claimed through 'genuine error'.

During my first year in training as a GP I got sick. I'd worked for many years in hospitals, had already qualified as a trainee in emergency medicine, but the intensity and breadth of problems I was learning to face in my new role as a doctor in the community felt to me overwhelming. An old recurrent problem with my sinuses flared up, leaving me with a ceaseless, drilling headache above and behind the eyes that sapped all of my energy. An MRI scan showed that I needed surgery, which might take months to arrange. In the meantime I had my GP training to complete.

I couldn't do anything to hurry up the arrival of my operation date, but I could do something about my exhaustion and my levels of stress. Rather than stop work altogether, I dropped to a three-day week – each day in clinic would be followed by a day off to recover. The headache was as bad as ever, but with more time to rest and recuperate between clinic days, the pain bothered me less. Knowing I'd have the breathing space of a day at home meant that I was able to give my best to my patients on those days I was in the clinic. My training would be delayed – it would now take longer than a year for me to be signed off as a competent GP – but I persuaded myself that there was no point risking burnout for the sake of sticking to a schedule of someone else's making.

And I qualified all the same, albeit a couple of months late. The operation, when it came, was successful, my headaches were cured, and I had learned a valuable lesson. We need strength and energy to live with illness; reducing my workload gave me the reserves I needed not just to live with chronic pain, but to begin on the path towards recovery from it.

Archaeologists who study the bones of our distant ancestors tell us that there was no golden age – for most of human history, most people worked hard all their lives and died young. Their bones are ridged with the attachments of strong muscles, their joints worn away by toil. Many were lucky to reach the age of forty. By the Victorian era it was proclaimed that charity began at home, but at the same time an anxiety took root that generosity bred idleness and corruption. Even the sick had to work for their keep – charitable provision was modest and was delivered through 'workhouses' or 'almshouses' where life expectancy was shockingly low.

Many of the patients I sign off from the obligation to find a job could undoubtedly work in some capacity, at something, if support were available to help them to do it. And work aids recovery in all sorts of ways, granting through physical and mental effort a sense of purpose, satisfaction and social connection, as well as a livelihood. If I could sign my patients up to a supportive back-to-work scheme, rather than simply signing them off sick, I would. But the truth is, the kind of support that is needed to help bring many people back into work is more expensive than the system of sickness benefits, and so there's little incentive for governments to pursue it.

If we aspire to a more civilised and

compassionate society than the one of Victorian workhouses, then we have to accept that the issue of who can work and who can't isn't just a question of objective tests, but one of compassion, society and culture.

Convalescence needs time, and the value we place on that time ultimately comes down to what our politicians will support. We are better at providing sickness benefits than we used to be – the half-century between 1945 and 1995 saw UK spending on sickness benefits increase ninefold – but there is still a long way to go to provide a truly supportive welfare safety net that allows everyone, rich or poor, to recover to the best of their capacity. There are many politicians who see today's modestly increased provision of benefits as evidence of a sick society, but I prefer to take it as heartening evidence that we are slowly (too slowly!) becoming a more compassionate society. Neither are UK payments to support sickness absence an unsustainable drain on the state, as is sometimes claimed.

These payments are regularly demonised in

the tabloid press, but they make up less than 0.002 per cent of the sum that was paid out to banks following the financial crash of 2008. It's another idiosyncrasy of sickness certification that its rules are set in legal terms, thrashed out in parliament or the courts in an adversarial environment that is profoundly at odds with the collaborative nature of medical consultations. And the alternative to this kind of provision would be to tolerate widespread destitution as a result of illness.

The politician Aneurin Bevan, who was pivotal in creating the UK's National Health Service, championed the idea that illness is 'neither an indulgence for which people have to pay nor an offence for which they should be penalised, but a misfortune the cost of which should be shared by the community'. This quote didn't actually come from the mouth of Bevan, but was written by a sociologist called T. H. Marshall as a summary of the guiding principles of the welfare state. It has been widely shared and repeated because at heart we recognise its truth: illness is not just a personal calamity, but a social one too; helping ease its effects is something we all must take a part in, as a community.

I've often wished that we could bring back into common use the term 'nervous breakdown' – a folk diagnosis capacious, vague, dramatic and elastic enough that it can be used in all sorts of situations. It can reinforce for people the gravity of the crisis they have found themselves in but avoids labelling them with a psychiatric diagnosis that might prove difficult to shake off. It can help them to take the appropriate time to recover. Recovery times vary from person to person, situation to situation – something that's as true for recovery from a breakdown in mental health as it is from a broken leg or from pneumonia.

It's not unusual for me to listen to the difficulties someone is having at work, and then to their list of symptoms – from sleeplessness to muscle pain, headaches to exhaustion – and to conclude: 'your work is making you sick.' I've known unscrupulous companies who gauge how hard to push their employees by simply charting office sickness rates – targets are piled on until sickness rates hit a certain threshold, and only then will the managers ease off the pressure. Modern call centres are so generative of anxiety and stress that they have 75 per cent higher turnover of staff than comparable office environments. I have many patients who work in such centres (often for those very banks that were the recipients of taxpayer generosity just over a decade ago). While some are generous, conscientious employers, others are exploitative.

Breakdowns in mental health, whether it be depressed mood, mania or debilitating anxiety, can often be triggered by such a work environment. There's even a ready-made code in healthcare's computer systems that is applied to sickness certificates given in such circumstances: *R007z* Work Stress. One study, by the Yale psychiatrists Paul B. Lieberman and John S. Strauss, called this kind of stress the 'enforced pursuit of an activity that was at odds with [a patient's] own goals and aspirations'.

*

I began medical training in the 1990s; the previous fifty years had seen the range of problems brought to the doors of GPs increase exponentially. Treatments such as antibiotics, steroids, chemotherapies and inhalers became so effective that people began to look to doctors for similarly dramatic cures for many of the other difficulties in their lives – difficulties not nearly so amenable to treatment by pills. My GP training began in a community of social and economic deprivation, and I remember the doctors there reminding me that for some of my patients, sickness certification could be the most important prescription I ever wrote. That attitude was summed up in a book of the period, *Doctors Talking*, which reproduced a series of anonymised interviews with GPs from communities across Scotland: island and city, wealthy and deprived. One of the GPs who worked in a particularly deprived inner city practice said:

Dealing with the links between poverty and ill health by trying to provide more money is no different, to me, from seeing a patient with pneumonia and prescribing antibiotics: in each situation, I'm simply giving appropriate treatment. Just as certain medicines are appropriate treatments for particular diseases, so more money, or holidays, or a better house, may also improve my patient's health.

Working to diminish social inequalities is a large part of relieving suffering – something far more in the gift of politicians than it is of doctors – but what doctors *can* sometimes do is to offer permission to take the time needed for recovery. It all depends on what you think of as medicine, and whether you consider the doctor as charged with the dispensing of pills or with the relief of suffering. I know which one I'd prefer.

The Hungarian psychoanalyst Michael Balint wrote 'falling ill, and especially being ill, is felt by many conscientious people as defaulting, demanding unfair advantages'. Balint was active and writing through the 1940s and 1950s, and his books are full of the casual bigotry of his age, making me wonder what prejudices and preconceptions of my own time will infuriate readers of the future. But for all the jarring statements, there are moments of deep wisdom in his writing. He did a great deal of work to understand the nature of the difficulties that people bring to their GPs, and noted that the majority fear being seen as inadequate, malingering or weak in seeking help: 'they feel guilty about getting more attention than seems fair to them, about not working, about living on someone else, and so on,' he wrote. For Balint, the true malingerer (defined as someone who'd fake illness because they believed it would give them an advantage in life) was rare: 'the type who is out to get more than his fair share, to whom any semblance of illness is more than welcome, who goes out of his way to "catch" diseases.' As a psychoanalyst, what interested Balint was that in his view both these kinds of convalescents, the industrious *and* the indolent, were troubled with self-reproach. 'Both of these types feel guilty, though for different reasons, and it is extremely difficult to get them better if the doctor cannot do something about their guilt feelings.'

Self-compassion is a much underrated virtue, and the rhythms of modern life are often antithetical to those of recovery. As workers in what we're so often told is a struggling economy, many of my patients feel a great deal of pressure to be maximally productive so as not to be a 'burden'. A century and a half ago economists and philosophers began to predict that, thanks to machines and mechanisation, humanity would have the opportunity to enjoy unprecedented prosperity and leisure. That has not been the experience of most. One of the most celebrated was Bertrand Russell, whose essay 'In Praise of Idleness' concluded:

Modern methods of production have given us the possibility of ease and security for all; we have chosen instead to have overwork for some and starvation for others. Hitherto we have continued to be as energetic as we were before there were machines. In this we have been foolish, but there is no reason to go on being foolish for ever.

The pressure to be maximally productive is learned early, and it can be a challenge to unpick inherited notions of what constitutes a successful life. But if we don't modify those ideas, we are unlikely to make time for recovery, or understand the value of rest and recuperation.

Oliver Sacks's *Gratitude* is not a book about convalescence per se, but about the expansion of consciousness that can be offered by illness, and Sacks's gradual reconciliation to a cancer that was slowly killing him. As his illness progressed, Sacks found himself thinking about what constitutes a good and worthwhile life – what the Greeks would have called *eudaemonia*, or 'flourishing', rather than simply the aspects of life that render it liveable.

To flourish we have to build in moments of rest and reflection. The Bengali poet Rabindranath Tagore summarised this sentiment when he wrote: 'in the rhythm of life, pauses there must be for the renewal of life. Life in its activity is ever spending itself, burning all its fuel.' Most people can identify with Tagore's observation, and will remember an experience of feeling as if they're all out of fuel, 'running on empty', needing to 'recharge the battery'. It's a vivid, immediately identifiable image, and I've often used the metaphor of the car or phone battery when discussing convalescence.

In one of the essays in *Gratitude*, Sacks explained how key for him in recovery was a sense of harmony and tranquillity. He felt a sense of peace when he came to accept the need for a kind of institutional or enforced rest 'when one can feel that one's work is done, and may, in good conscience, rest'. That 'good conscience' is telling: Sacks struggled to give himself the permission to rest until he was approaching the end of his life and was undergoing treatment for malignant melanoma. He began to embrace the necessity of taking some kind of rest every seventh day – an ancient concept enshrined in the concept of the 'sabbath' (Hebrew for 'seventh'). The workplace has formalised the need for this kind of refuelling, or recharging the battery, with the 'sabbatical'.

The original sabbaticals were a Near Eastern tradition in which every seventh year a wealthy (invariably male) householder was expected to release all of his slaves, leave his land untilled, and go on a journey or religious pilgrimage. The sabbatical was a social institution that enforced a break from routine and from the pressures of work, in order to be able to facilitate the possibility of returning to it renewed. To journey away from the familiar has always been one of the best-travelled roads through convalescence.

We could all do with a sabbatical from time to time, though a year off every seventh might seem extreme. In my own GP practice, my colleagues and I have formalised a compromise into our contracts as a three-month break every five years. I return from my own sabbaticals relaxed, reinspired, and energised by the time away. I can't rewrite my patients' employment contracts to make sure that they can access sabbaticals, but I can encourage them to find ways to try.

5

TRAVEL

A change is as good as a rest, they say, and since the time of Hippocrates, convalescents have been urged to get away on holiday. I recommend one as often as I can, and have heard that in Sweden and Finland, it's even possible to prescribe holidays at the taxpayer's expense (for the treatment of psoriasis – apparently it's cheaper and more effective to send people from Scandinavia on a sunny holiday than it is to pay for inpatient hospital treatment with ultraviolet light). The Roman statesman Cicero said that the doctors of his day often recommended a change of place for those in convalescence: 'very often the cure is effected by change of place, as sick people, that have not recovered their strength, are benefited by change of air.' The principle is that if something isn't working, then change it: sometimes we need change and new air, new experiences, and new reflections to jolt us out of unhelpful habits of mind. Darwin noted that this universal truth of life appeared to apply not only to humans but to animals and plants, even to seeds and tubers when transferred from one climate to another by farmers.

During the Middle Ages those who suffered poor health often undertook pilgrimages, primarily with a religious motive, and any benefit accrued from the journey was often ascribed to divine intervention rather than to the change of scene. Chaucer's *Canterbury Tales* sets out healing as one of the principal motives of his pilgrims: 'And specially, from every shire's end Of England, to Canterbury they wend, The holy blissful Martyr for to seek, Who helped them when they were sick.' The challenges of travelling for weeks on end by foot or horse-back must have been considerable – the words 'travel' and 'travail' have the same root – and in the case of longer journeys many of the frailer pilgrims must have died on the way. But for those who successfully managed to complete a distant pilgrimage, the reaching of a spiritual goal, and the sense of accomplishment from having triumphed through such an ordeal, must have been of profound benefit to both body and mind. It's also hard to think of a more convincing placebo than a quest to behold a magical or spiritual object, about which you've already heard many testimonials of cure.

Many years ago now, one of my own sceptical patients went on pilgrimage to Lourdes at his daughter's request. He was dying of cancer, and on his return to my clinic it was clear that the progress of his disease had continued unabated. But he didn't regret the journey: his arrival at the shrine, and the experience of being surrounded by a community of other pilgrims, had felt as valuable to him as any of my morphine prescriptions.

The journey or pilgrimage takes us away from the local and particular circumstances of our illness, and the factors that surround its onset: sometimes this is enough to cause the illness to simply melt away. To embark on a journey we often have to throw aside the obligations of life, and in that moment of abandonment it becomes possible to see more clearly which of those obligations are truly dispensable, which should be restored, and how it might be best to rearrange them, if at all, when we return. But even in cases where the illness sticks stubbornly to the body or mind, a long journey or holiday offers new perspectives and strategies with which to live in renewed reconciliation with a condition.

And just as road trips can be therapeutic, so can journeys out of ourselves through the pages of books. Jack Kerouac's *On the Road* sees the book's narrator Sal Paradise assert that while divorce had freed him to travel, his journey was justified as a form of convalescence ('I had just gotten over a serious illness'), and for more than sixty years Kerouac's book has been used as a kind of vicarious journey of liberation for the armchair traveller. For those of us who can't be prescribed a foreign holiday, time spent in recovery can be repetitive and dreary, and as a convalescent it's easy to feel trapped. Books can unlock the sick room door on to somewhere more expansive and free.

Of the restorative value of books, J. R. R. Tolkien wrote in *Tree and Leaf* that reading acts 'as a holiday, and a refreshment. It is splendid for convalescence; and not only for that, for many it is the best introduction to the Mountains. It works wonders in some cases.' It's a beautiful idea: books as our seaways and railways, our trails and tracks, carrying us with them on a journey of recovery.

6

THE ARCHITECTURE OF RECOVERY

For wealthy people it was once common for a period of convalescence to take in time at a sanatorium, spa or convalescent hospital. These were spaces designed for the benefit and comfort of patients, not staff. These days the contract for new hospitals is put out to tender, and architects compete to come up with the cheapest design. New hospitals often have much in common with airports and supermarkets: low plastic ceilings, little natural light, retail forecourts, windows that don't open, and views, where they exist, giving on to car parks rather than the green space so beloved of Florence Nightingale.

The exception is modern hospices for the terminally ill, which almost uniquely retain the concerns of the old convalescent hospitals with gardens, space, quiet, and natural light. But, by chance, two of the Edinburgh hospitals where I undertook my own medical training were once convalescent hospitals. The first, the Princess Margaret Rose, was built high on a bluff to the south of the city, its patios and wide windows angled to make the most of weak Scottish sunshine, as well as blasts of air from the Pentland Hills. I remember doing rounds as a medical student in those light-filled wards, listening to the wind rattling the windows. It was first intended as a hospital for tuberculosis patients, back in the years when the only treatment for tuberculosis was time, clean air and rest (though occasionally they also collapsed your worst-affected lung, to starve the tuberculosis bacilli of oxygen). With the coming of antibiotics the tuberculosis hospitals have all closed, but with their demise, we have lost something of value. In Switzerland some of the old sanatoriums have been converted to hospital units concerned with other long-term illnesses not amenable to quick-fix solutions: mental health, alcoholism, drug-dependency. Each of those have their own journeys of recovery.

At the time of my training, the Princess Margaret Rose was used solely for orthopaedic surgery. Many of the patients I saw there had been broken in bone then remade with titanium pins and plates; all benefited from the humane and thoughtful architecture of the traditional TB hospital – all on one level, with wide corridors to permit wheelchair-manoeuvres, and those glorious sunlit south-facing wards. It was a reminder too of a time when prime real estate was kept aside for the sick. Like so many old hospitals, it has now been knocked down and replaced with sought-after luxury housing.

The other convalescent hospital where I was taught is still going – for the moment at least. The foundation of the Astley Ainslie Hospital is described in the Lothian Health Archives like this:

Mr David Ainslie of Costerton, Midlothian, died in 1900 leaving instructions to his trustees that the residue of his estate, after a lapse of 15 years, was to be applied 'to the purpose of erecting, endowing and maintaining a hospital or institution to be called the Astley Ainslie Institution, for the relief and behoof of the convalescents of the Royal Infirmary of Edinburgh'.

Four mansions were purchased – Millbank, Southbank, Canaan House and Canaan Park – and the hospital was opened in 1923. Over the subsequent decade a series of whitewashed pavilions were built between the mansions, each surrounded by arboreal lanes, trimmed lawns, and weedless flower beds. At that time the city's main hospital, the Royal Infirmary, had a dedicated 'convalescent unit' in the west of the city at Corstorphine, but the patients who needed even longer-term care and recuperation than was available there were moved to the Astley Ainslie. The health archives also note that the Astley Ainslie 'might also take in Royal Infirmary patients who needed to be built up for surgery'. Imagine: a hospital that would not only look after people until they were strong enough to be 'fit for normal life', but would also take people in *before* surgery, to get them as fit as they could be. In the 1940s and 1950s Edinburgh provided so many convalescent hospital beds that they came under a separate board of management. It's more than half a century since we've had such a board because we no longer value that kind of convalescence.

Today, the Astley Ainslie Hospital is still concerned with recovery, in its way – it is a haven of rest and recuperation for those disabled by injury or by neurological conditions such as strokes or multiple sclerosis. Its physiotherapists outnumber its doctors. But it is also under threat: when it is sold off for housing, and its patients moved out to a modern facility, we will have done the people of Edinburgh (and Mr David Ainslie) a great disservice.

7

THE REST CURE

I like to imagine Dr Silas Weir Mitchell, who was by 1900 the president of Philadelphia's College of Physicians, as the archetypal doctor of the later nineteenth century. Perhaps on his rounds he'd wear a top hat and tails, and a tight-buttoned waistcoat into which he'd nestle a watch on a gold chain, his medical bag for those private patients one of polished leather. He was a neurologist in the years when there was no distinction between disorders of the brain and of the mind, and was a great advocate of what he called the 'Rest Cure'. This was prescribed for what was at the time termed 'neurasthenia', or 'weak nerves' in which people were to be encouraged to spend months at a time in bed, eating what he called a 'blood and fat' diet. Virginia Woolf ridiculed his ideas in *Mrs Dalloway*: '[you] order rest in bed; rest in solitude; silence and rest; rest without friends, without books, without messages; six months' rest; until a man who went in weighing seven stone six comes out weighing twelve.'

Women were recommended this treatment far more often than men. In a short story called 'The Yellow Wallpaper', one of America's earliest feminist writers, Charlotte Perkins Gilman, laid bare the way the medical establishment was using the excuse of these 'cures' to imprison people against their will: in effect forcing un-cooperative women into a weaker and more passive role. It's a role that still influences the way convalescents are seen today. The story of Weir Mitchell's 'Rest Cure' is a reminder of the power doctors have over us to define how we see ourselves, and how we are perceived. His advice is remembered today as emblematic of a certain kind of misogyny then prevalent in medicine, and which we have yet to entirely shake off.

To spend months in bed simply eating and sleeping might sound perfect for a healing body or mind, but Weir Mitchell's advice was medically inadvisable: it risks the melting of muscle from bones, and the withering of connections that sustain social lives. We are gregarious beings who need to act in the world, and any idea of convalescence that doesn't take this into account is doomed to fail.

When a patient of mine has pneumonia I prescribe a course of antibiotics for a week (two if there's a degree of chronic lung damage), and discuss the advice I was taught on the wards: to keep well hydrated, breathe deeply, and rest propped up in bed so that gravity can help your diaphragm to fill the lungs fully with air. I tell those convalescents that even with antibiotics every decade you've lived may add a week to your recovery time from such an infection – a couple of months for someone in their eighties. Phlegm and mucus will continue to be coughed up from the lungs for some time after the antibiotics are finished, but this is all part of healing – the lining of the lung renewing itself. Despite those warnings, however, many are still surprised when, at the end of their antibiotic prescription, they don't feel entirely well.

Flawed though it was, Weir Mitchell's advice still has some value for us, given how much he emphasised the importance of giving adequate time to recovery. In the pre-antibiotic era, even young, fit patients would take at least a month to get over the worst initial crisis of pneumonia – a month in which it wasn't unusual for them to lose a quarter of their body weight through recurrent, wringing fevers. Weir Mitchell described this loss as the 'debt to disease'. But alongside that loss sat an equivalent gain or resurgence of life force: illness was imagined as a kind of struggle with death, a perennial *memento mori* from which we would emerge as if reborn. He wrote: 'Millions of dead molecules are being restored in such better condition that not only are you become new in the best sense – renewed, as we say, – but have gotten power to grow again.'

Recovery had other 'amiable' aspects, according to Weir Mitchell: it was a potentially valuable time of liberation from work and family commitments. 'One feels at peace with all the world, and so lies still, and reflects as to whether, on the whole, the matter has not had its valuable side.'

In addition to the 'Rest Cure', Weir Mitchell became famous for another approach to recovery, dubbed the 'West Cure' (and the 'West' was as much a product of its time as the 'Rest'). It was recommended far more often to men suffering from neurasthenia than it was to women suffering the same. Recipients would be advised to journey to the Midwest, and seek work on a ranch or in the mountains where they would be obliged to sleep on the ground, herd steers or cut down trees. The 'West Cure' had adherents from Teddy Roosevelt to Walt Whitman, all of whom spent time through the 1870s and 1880s 'out west', specifically as a cure for what was thought to be weak nerves.

It was a mistake to position these two modes of convalescence, 'Rest' and 'West', as mutually exclusive when they so clearly had the same goal – to help someone, anyone, recover health and strength. Rather than separating activity and resting – let alone doing so by gender – it's a combination of the two, in my experience, that is a more helpful approach for everyone. A greater respect for the importance of rest can coexist with an understanding of how vital it is that we remain active and engaged in the world.

In an essay for the American Psychological Association, the literary scholar Anne Stiles pointed out just how much Weir Mitchell's ideas are still part of medical ideas of convalescence, in an age when 'over-stressed business executives of both sexes travel to pristine natural destinations in search of relaxation and self-discovery, sometimes combined with rigorous physical activities, such as biking or mountaineering'. That both men and women are now encouraged to 'go west' in search of recovery surely speaks of some kind of progress, just as both may well benefit from accepting the need for rest. But it's not only high-powered professionals who can benefit from a change of scene and a focus on a more natural environment.

Activity is good for us – there's an entire professional discipline dedicated to 'occupational therapy' after all – but there seems to be something particularly powerful about the kind of natural settings Weir Mitchell had in mind. Some years ago now, a young man with a job in computing attended my clinic every fortnight or so with a new symptom: headaches, knee pain, itching rashes, throat tightness. He felt as if his bladder was never entirely empty, then that it could never get entirely full. Whenever I started to get an understanding of one of his symptoms his principal complaint would shift and I'd have to start all over again with a new one. It was clear that, more than a cure, what he sought was acknowledgement of his suffering.

I began to explore this with him, pointing out how often his symptoms shifted and how that was frequently the sign of an underlying malaise, unhappiness, or stress in the circumstances of his life rather than some bodily problem. I wondered whether there was something that deep down he knew he needed to change about the way he was living his life.

One day, he didn't turn up for his appointment. That in itself wasn't unusual, but when I didn't hear from him for many months I wondered whether I'd done something to offend. I asked the receptionists whether he'd gone off my list, shifting to another doctor elsewhere, but no – he was still on the books of my practice.

When he did get in touch, it was by postcard: a snowy mountain scene, forests, a river running through the foreground and, on that river, a flotilla of kayaks. Beneath the picture was the name of an activity centre in the Scottish Highlands, and scribbled on the back were words suggesting that he'd found his own balance between 'rest' and 'west'. 'Dear Dr Francis,' it said, 'I've been working up here all year and they've offered me a permanent job. The new rhythm suits me, so thanks for your help, but I don't think I'll be coming back.'

8

BACK TO NATURE

All worthwhile acts of recovery have to work in concert with natural processes, not against them: antibiotics in the class of penicillin do not 'kill' bacteria, they merely arrest the growth of bacterial colonies and leave the body to do the rest. A doctor who sets out to 'heal' is in truth more like a gardener who sets out to 'grow' – actually, nature does almost all of the work. Even when I stitch a patient's wound the suture material itself does not knit the tissues – that thread is simply a trellis to guide the body in its own work of recovery.

For Renaissance artists and anatomists there was little distinction between art and science: both were ways of celebrating and understanding the truth about the world. They also saw a continuity between the body we inhabit and the environment that sustains us. Many traditional approaches to medicine, before the rise of science, saw the body as embedded within and reflecting the cosmos: the environment around us held the key to restitution. Medicine in ancient Greece depended on dietary regimens and finding an optimal climate. Illness was a disturbance in the elements that the body shared with the universe – the four elements of matter were in correspondence with the four 'humours' that sustained life. That perspective was still going strong by the sixteenth century. Leonardo da Vinci wrote: 'If a man is made of earth, water, air and fire, so is this body of the earth; if man has in him a lake of blood ... the body of the earth has its ocean, which similarly rises and falls.'

When taken too far, the idea of redressing natural balance between the inner and outer environments can lead to dangerous quackery – to advocating crystal therapy against leukaemia or reflexology against septicaemia. But the extraordinary success of scientific medicine risks divorcing the body from ideas of the environment that nourishes us. That we are animals, part of life, caught between growth and entropy, was something beautifully explored by Thomas Mann in his great novel of convalescence, *The Magic Mountain*, which sees its hero lying in a sanatorium high in the Alps, considering the nature of illness and recovery:

> What then was life? ... It was the existence of the actually impossible-to-exist, of a half-sweet, half-painful balancing, or scarcely balancing, in this restricted and feverish process of decay and renewal, upon the point of existence. It was not matter and it was not spirit, but something between the two, a phenomenon conveyed by matter, like the rainbow on the waterfall, and like the flame.

This idea of the body as belonging to the green organic world of Life is something often forgotten in the clinics and hospital wards where I've trained and worked in medicine, so much so that it came as a surprise to read of a physician who has taken it to the heart of her clinical management. Dr Victoria Sweet is an associate professor of medicine at the University of California, San Francisco, with a PhD in the medieval history of medicine. For many years she worked in one of the last almshouses in the United States – a hospital for the poor who have nowhere else to go.

In her book *God's Hotel* Sweet describes how, after years of reading about the medieval nun and healer Hildegard of Bingen, she came to the conclusion that to better describe the aims of recovery we should resurrect Hildegard's medieval concept of *viriditas*, or 'greening'. To be healed is to be reinvigorated by the same force that animates trees as much as it does human beings, and the work of the physician is much more like that of a gardener than it is like a mechanic. She came to realise that the 'rule of fours' – four elements of matter, four seasons, four humours, four 'qualities' (hot, wet, cold and dry) – used by physicians for over two thousand years was still on occasion a fruitful way of looking at the body and its needs. If something is too cold then warm it, too dry then wet it, and so on. It's a gardener's view, as well as a doctor's, because it holds at the centre of its vision that concept of balance – health as the equilibrium between extremes, rather than an end in itself to be 'reached' or 'achieved'.

This makes intuitive sense: until very recently physicians had to study botany, not only because so many medicines are derived from plants, but because the study of plants is a way to understand life itself. The GP I had as a child, the one who sent me urgently to hospital with meningitis, told me later that he had to take botany classes as part of his Edinburgh Medical School curriculum in the 1950s. Again, it is as if with the pharmaceutical revolutions of the later twentieth century we've forgotten something of the importance of a broader approach to recovery. Sweet describes Hildegard's attendance on the sick as comparable in its approach to her work in the convent garden. Convalescence was led by the same principles, and she thought about the body's response to nutrients, to light and water, to rest and exercise, in the same way as she thought about helping plants to grow.

The word 'physician' can be rooted back to the Greek *physis*, meaning 'nature', and *phuo*, which means 'to grow'. Just like a plant, what we need in order to grow back into wholeness is a 'regime' of the right nutrients, the right environment, the right resources, and to be undisturbed – what Sweet summarises as 'Dr Diet, Dr Quiet, and Dr Merryman'.

Today all that we have left of regime is the monotonous injunctions to lose weight, lower our cholesterol, sleep eight hours a day, exercise, and be cheerful. Hildegard and premodern medicine were more subtle. Nothing was bad or good but as it suited the season, the climate, and the person. So she might recommend beer to fatten up the anorexic and forbid red wine to the choleric;

in spring, fresh green shoots were good; in winter, stews. For the love-sick, distraction; for the scattered and anxious, focus.

This attitude to recovery has been crowded out in modern medicine because it takes time. Sweet wrote another book, called *Slow Medicine*, to emphasise how, in the race to cut inpatient hospital time (and by extension in her US context, save money and expand profits), any emphasis on the value of slow recovery has been discarded. Sweet wouldn't want to return to medieval medicine, and wouldn't give up our blood tests and scans, our robotic surgery or antibiotics. But she would like to see the value of time restored to the practice of medicine. And so would I.

9

THE IDEAL DOCTOR

The great Canadian physician William Osler wrote that 'It is much more important to know what sort of patient has the disease than to know what sort of disease the patient has'. To that I might add 'and equally important to know what kind of physician each patient needs'. Doctors bring their own personalities and experience to every medical encounter, and we know that people recover more quickly from physical conditions if they perceive their doctor as sympathetic to their concerns. Psychological research into 'compassion fatigue' has shown that medical students begin their studies with a great deal of compassion, but the longer they work in the profession, the more they seem to lose it. We need to do better as a profession to keep our doctors from burnout, but I also think it's a mistake to characterise empathy as a fixed quality of the personality, which each student or doctor possesses to a greater or lesser degree. My own experience of empathy and compassion in medicine is as something far more dynamic and alive: a state of understanding and connection between two people. Some doctors are undoubtedly more open to this kind of connection than others, but it remains a two-way process – not a solo but a duet.

The GP and writer John Launer tells the story of a patient who announced, even as she was sitting down in his consulting room, 'I've got three problems.' The way the UK health services are funded means that GPs have about ten minutes allocated for each patient and so Launer had just three minutes to address each of his patient's concerns. Launer didn't miss a beat, but replied 'And what's the fourth?' In his book *How Not to Be a Doctor* he explains how the rest of the consultation went: '[the fourth] was the problem that she both dreaded and desperately wanted to tell me, and we never got back to the original three problems.'

The word 'doctor' comes from the Latin *docere*, meaning 'to teach' or 'to guide', and just as every teacher you've ever had works with a different style, so do doctors. The idea that there's a universal approach within any branch of medicine is false, and would be a terrible way to offer medical care. Launer was working with his intuition, not his medical training, and on that occasion his hunch paid off. But hunches can just as easily be wrong: in the thirty or forty medical encounters I have in the course of a normal working day there must be several that I misjudge, guessing wrongly which kind of doctor that particular patient needs me to be.

The kind of intuition that Launer is talking about isn't something that can be taught. What can be taught is the confidence to act on the small voices of conscience and experience that suggest when a therapeutic relationship will benefit from going off-piste – away from the well-trimmed paths of textbook solutions into something wilder and more unscripted.

The psychoanalyst and paediatrician Donald Winnicott thought that doctors should become familiar with what he called the 'mechanisms' of human psychology, but not *too* familiar, lest they lose 'spontaneity and intuitive understanding'; for Winnicott, physicians act best on intuition, rather than on what textbooks have told them to do. Within modern medicine this creates a conflict, between an idea of a clinical encounter that should be measurable, reproducible and thus open to professional regulation of standards, and the idea of a clinical encounter as the unique alchemy between two human beings that combines the experience of each in an unrepeatable moment that changes both of them.

Doctors must be well grounded in the science of medicine – that isn't up for debate. But what is open to question is whether scientific knowledge is where medical practice ends, or where it begins. The answer might of course be different for different people. I have some patients who see me solely as the conduit through which to gain access to specialists, and others who want from me, as a representative of the scientific establishment, only the facts of their particular condition. And at the other end of the spectrum I've known patients for whom the aim of our consultations is to feel cared for, and to be given a sense of confidence in their recovery even when their condition is one that can't be cured.

'The confidence (or lack of) which a doctor feels about a patient's recovery can affect the outcome of their illness,' wrote Jay Griffiths of her GP, whom she met repeatedly throughout a breakdown in her mental health. Griffiths' GP offered continual reassurance that had its origin in his deep knowledge of her as someone he'd seen recover before, and of having seen so many others recover over the years. '"You're going to be okay, you're going to be okay," was unforgettable as a spell,' Griffiths wrote. 'It engendered belief in me and that belief went a long way to working its own cure.'

For Griffiths, to have been given solely the

facts of her condition would have done her a disservice, just as it would have been a disservice for John Launer to quietly listen to his patient's three irrelevant problems. Understanding the body and its failings is the easiest part of medicine. Knowing what kind of doctor each patient needs is far more difficult.

Many years ago I worked with a GP who recognised that sometimes the most helpful thing she could do was to listen to, and acknowledge, her patients' stories of suffering. As she listened to those stories she'd place her hands over her stomach, fingers interlaced, as a kind of symbolic shield. 'That way the emotions in the room don't settle on me,' she explained. 'With my hands there to protect me, they bounce off.' I knew another GP who worked abroad in a language of which he had only a modest grasp. His poor understanding of his patients' words should have made it almost impossible to practise medicine, but he told me he was very popular, and had tremendous results. 'I understand only about half of what they're saying,' he told me; 'but they really seem to appreciate that I'm listening so carefully.' I remember a long consultation with someone recovering slowly from a post-viral fatigue. It was a conversation in which I hardly spoke, and I was surprised, at the end, to be told how helpful I'd been. 'I didn't say anything,' I said as we walked towards the exit. 'But you listened,' she replied.

When we bring our hope of recovery to a doctor we may not be certain whether to focus on the biology of our illness or on its biography, but either can work as a way into a deeper understanding of how we have arrived at the crisis that has brought us to the consulting room. Biology and biography are equally valid ways of understanding illness. As John Launer writes, 'GPs work permanently on the knife edge between diagnosis of illness and the interpretation of experience.' Just as some people need to understand the science of their disease in order to better appreciate how to defeat it, others need to understand illness as a story that is tending towards a happy ending.

*

For some people, being offered groundless reassurances is irritating. When he was dying of prostate cancer the literary critic Anatole Broyard didn't want a physician who would treat him with too much respect, tiptoeing around his feelings, but someone who'd joke with him, cajole him, tell him to keep his chin up and get on with it, and not offer false comfort. He also wrote about the kind of doctors he liked best: bookish ones. 'St Luke was a doctor: Imagine having Chekhov, who was a doctor, for your doctor. Imagine having William Carlos Williams, who was a poet, or Walker Percy, who's a novelist, for your doctor. Imagine having Rabelais, who was a doctor, as your physician. My God, I could conjure with him!' One of the doctors he saw seemed to him too meek and polite to 'prevail over something powerful and demonic like illness'. Another he mentions was too much of a maverick, 'a sort of Donald Trump of critical illness ... he reminds me of a doctor I knew who wore such outlandish-looking suits that I couldn't help wondering about his medical judgment'. For

Broyard, the ideal physician was an almost impossibly august, well-balanced and well-read figure, capable of being a critic of medicine just as Broyard had been a critic of literature: 'a talented physician, but a bit of a metaphysician, too'. And for all his dreams of the ideal doctor, he knew his expectations were unreasonable: 'The sick man asks far too much, he is *im*patient in everything, and his doctor may be afraid of making a fool of himself in trying to reply.' The best doctors use their intuition to gauge what kind of doctor each patient needs, but for some, those needs are so specific or inflated they are impossible to meet.

So what can we expect of our physicians? Doctors get accustomed to the disappointment of being unable to cure their patients; if a patient expects their doctor to heal every illness, they'll be disappointed too. I've always found it less damaging to think of myself as a guide rather than a healer, someone who in three decades of clinical practice has seen many different landscapes of human suffering, but who has never, and will never, have seen them all. My hope is to help patients across those landscapes of illness of which I have some knowledge, and, for those that are new to me, to call on what useful experience I can, as well as the expertise of others. Doctor-as-guide is an ancient idea: St Basil, a fourth-century saint in the eastern Mediterranean (said to have founded the first public hospital), said that we should call in doctors in the same way 'as we entrust the helm to the pilot in the art of navigation'.

Broyard knew that for a doctor, every day in clinic is a circuit of human suffering, while for the patient, what they bring to the doctor might represent the crisis of their life. It's something that was brought home to me most forcibly when I worked in an emergency department. Every fifteen minutes or so would bring an encounter that, for my patients, might be the most terrifying event of their year, their decade, or even of the whole of their lives. Most clinicians deal with the shock of this kind of exposure through a hardened retreat into a distanced professionalism – a retreat that can salvage their sanity. But for Broyard, a doctor who resisted that hardening, who maintained some softness or vulnerability to the stories of their patients, would be more than compensated for their trouble, and would gain immeasurably in their humanity.

It's to be celebrated that different doctors are different, and have different approaches to medicine and to recovery. If someone feels that they and their doctor are speaking separate languages, it might be worth changing for another, or at least acknowledging that there is a lack of understanding between them. No clinician wants to have ineffective consultations. But beware of swapping for the sake of it – whatever politicians might hope for, healthcare can never be a marketplace in any ordinary sense of the word. The stakes are too high, there is rarely the opportunity to compare like with like, and you have to have faith in a doctor (and their prescriptions) in a way that's not necessary with a shopkeeper. Medicine is nothing like shopping.

Over the course of my career I've encountered many occasions when a companionable approach to guiding a patient across the landscape of a new illness doesn't work. Relationships break down, the disease takes an unexpected turn, expectations of what is possible soar out of reach of what any physician or nurse would be capable of providing. The principal virtue of any therapeutic relationship is trust. When trust has gone, it becomes very difficult to heal.

10

WRITING YOUR OWN STORY

There's a passage in *Moby Dick* where the hero of the story, Ishmael, is lamenting the sickness of his dying friend Queequeg. Queequeg is a Polynesian harpoonist, unencumbered with American ideas of ill health and, by consequence, bodily recovery. Melville describes him as being so sure that he is about to die that he builds his own coffin and climbs in. Lying there on the verge of death, Queequeg remembers something important that he wishes to do ashore before he dies, and so promptly recovers.

His crewmates ask him then whether to live or to die is a matter of choice and will-power, to which he answers, 'certainly': 'it was

Queequeg's conceit, that if a man made up his mind to live, mere sickness could not kill him: nothing but a whale, or a gale, or some violent, ungovernable, unintelligent destroyer of that sort.'

It's a potent idea – that there are illnesses that can be overcome by power of the will, while there are others that are unassailable because of their violence, their 'ungovernable' capacity to destroy.

Our mental capacity to influence the renewal of health is formidable – it's what many believe powers the placebo effect. Recovery is in no way a matter of willpower as such, but it can on occasion be influenced by mental attitude all the same. The most tested drug in the world is the placebo, because every new medication has to be assessed in a trial against it, and what comes up in study after study is how astonishingly effective placebos are. The word itself means 'I will please', acknowledging that sometimes we need to feel as if we're taking control of an illness, influencing its outcome, whatever the true merits of the medication or intervention – a placebo helps us do just that. It's a fascinating aspect of placebos that their colour dictates their effectiveness: red, yellow and orange are more effective for deadening pain or acting as stimulants, while blue and green are more effective as sedatives. Capsule placebos work better than tablets.

And if placebos can cure us through manipulating our expectations, it's also true to say that our expectations are equally powerful in terms of making us ill.

Suzanne O'Sullivan is a neurologist in London specialising in what are now called 'functional illnesses' and used to be called 'psychosomatic' illnesses. Her books *It's All in Your Head* and *The Sleeping Beauties* describe many devastating disorders caused not by tumour or poisoning or infection or inflammation, but by complex interplay between shifting layers of biological, psychological and sociological meaning. It used to be thought that psychosomatic illnesses always had their origins in 'stress', a word imported into medicine from engineering, and which until relatively recently was used only to describe pressures applied to materials such as steel, wood or stone. But O'Sullivan has many patients who have experienced no particular stress in their lives. Their illnesses have arisen instead from their beliefs and expectations, by the same kind of mechanism that causes outbreaks of mass hysteria. Just as humans tend to believe that red pills are more powerful than white pills, what you believe about your illness has an immense impact on the way that you feel, and on the outcome.

I remember telephoning a patient of mine to tell him that his blood tests had demonstrated profound anaemia. He was out cycling at the time, and had already ridden a couple of miles without difficulty. But with the knowledge of his anaemia the whole experience of that ride changed, breathlessness came over him, and he became incapable of pedalling the couple of miles home. Another of my patients believed that an injury to her eye had rendered her blind on one side – the left. She had never learned that the anatomy of vision means that injuries to the eye affect the contrary field of vision, and so left-sided injuries cause disturbance of vision to the right. Her left-sided blindness was anatomically impossible, but nevertheless remained demonstrably *true for her*.

Beliefs about illness can be incredibly powerful, and deaths have been known to occur through expectation and, in a certain sense, through faith. O'Sullivan describes an epidemic of deaths among Hmong people from Laos who were given refugee status in the US through the 1970s and 1980s, and many of whom, finding their new home hostile and bewildering, began to die in their sleep. No biological explanation has ever been found, and O'Sullivan proposes that these deaths were in some way triggered through despair: 'The Hmong suggested that they had been terrorized to death by a nightmare,' O'Sullivan added; 'Nobody has ever offered a better explanation.'

I once worked in a small hospital in the Scottish Highlands where a woman was sent from her distant village on her seventieth birthday.

Her bemused GP had sent in a letter stating that the woman was convinced she was about to die, because scripture set her lifespan at threescore years and ten. Nothing he said could convince her otherwise. She was clerked into the hospital, assessed, deemed healthy, and transport home was arranged for the following day. But she *did* die, that same night, and at her post-mortem no explanation was found.

If only we could will ourselves back to health, as Queequeg willed himself out of his coffin. But recovery, of course, is rarely that simple. We can sometimes help it along by finding new understandings of our illness, by shifting our expectations and, through education, making a reappraisal of our beliefs. As an example of the latter, Suzanne O'Sullivan describes a patient who had become paralysed through a faulty understanding of anatomy: she believed that the 'slipped disc' in her back was cutting through her spinal cord. It was only with a thorough explanation of spinal anatomy (one of the reasons a plastic skeleton hangs in my consulting room) and with

a physiotherapist's skill and gentle encouragement, that the patient began to understand
that her slipped disc couldn't cut through her
spinal cord or paralyse her leg. Once her belief
was seen for what it was – a misunderstanding
– she began to recover.

Understanding the anatomy and the func-
tions of the body in this way can often help in
recovery, as can old-fashioned conjuring tricks:
amputees have been successfully treated for
the agonising condition of 'phantom limb' pain
through simply viewing their body in mirrors
that give the illusion that the operated limb has
been made whole.

We are complicated beings, made up of
mind and body. But we are also members of
communities of belief that influence the way
that we make sense of our symptoms. We
experience our bodies on many different levels,
and our feelings are influenced by our expectations. No one is suggesting that such healing
stories are easy to find, or once found that they
are straightforward to harness in the service of
health. From an understanding of the anatomy

of paralysis, to an acknowledgement of the reality of post-viral fatigue, for some conditions the best way towards recovery is to find a new story that makes sense of our experience, even if it's not always possible to give ourselves a fairy-tale ending. Accepting that different stories are even possible, and can be rewritten, is a powerful step in the right direction.

11

ON CARERS

On a children's ward in the tropics where I once worked, babies and toddlers with life-threatening malaria were cared for largely by their mothers, not by the overstretched nurses. The fevers these children suffered were so high they'd often trigger seizures, and to keep the body temperature down the nursing staff showed those mothers how to sponge down the children with tepid water. That vital work of supporting, feeding, washing and cooling often made the difference between life and death.

Some of us are lucky enough to have a memory of childhood illness that carries that sense of being looked after, of being *cared* for, an early experience of caring as a gentle act of love. And for many people young and old, that experience of being cared for is part of adulthood too. Through the Covid pandemic it has been estimated that, in the UK, unpaid carers saved the state the equivalent of half a billion pounds every day. Being able to care for a loved one feels like an essential aspect of our humanity, whether it's a life-saving intervention like those mothers on the malaria ward, or something more modest – a help into a wheelchair, a shave when you can't manage it, being brought soup in bed.

But care can also be exhausting for those who provide it: a carers' charity in my city, called Vocal, offers a series of educational and social events, afternoons and evenings, offering not just peer and emotional support, but practical, financial and even domestic help – overnight respite and help with getting away on holiday. There are many other such charities – Carers UK, Carers Trust, Age UK and the Alzheimer's Society, to name a few. Upcoming workshops when I checked the Vocal website recently for one of my own patients included advice on sleep problems, compassion fatigue, grief, information on particular disabilities, and the meeting details of a book club.

Carers' support has plummeted through the Covid pandemic lockdowns, and I've seen the lives of my patients suffer enormously as a result: children with special needs, adults with physical disabilities and people living with dementia all struggled with the widespread closure of support services that were instituted, after all, as support for carers as much as for patients themselves. In my daily work as a GP, charged with supporting carers, sometimes all I can do is to offer a sympathetic ear and make a call to one of those charities. I wish I could do more.

Sometimes becoming a carer involves a complete transformation of life. In 1999 the journalist Allan Little was working in Moscow as the BBC's Russia correspondent when his partner Sheena McDonald, then living in London, was injured in a road traffic accident.

She sustained a severe head injury, was rendered immediately unconscious, and by the time Allan heard of the accident she was on a ventilator in intensive care.

He flew to London within hours of hearing the news, and for two weeks sat at her bedside in University College Hospital's intensive care unit, then again at her bedside in the brain injury unit of London's specialist hospital for neurology in Queen Square, for five more weeks. But as is so often the case with convalescence, the real difficulties of recovery began once Sheena was well enough to be discharged home. In the book they wrote together along with the neuropsychologist Gail Robinson, *Rebuilding Life after Brain Injury*, Allan writes movingly about the critical but underacknowledged role that partners, parents, children and carers necessarily play in any convalescent's recovery. It's an extraordinary book: a narrative of brain injury by someone who has recovered from it, an intimate testimony by the partner of someone in recovery, and a clinical guidebook on how it's possible to help someone recover to their fullest potential following such an injury.

Injury to the brain is particularly pernicious in that it attacks memory, vitality, social behaviour, mood and the capacity for language, all at once. A huge amount is asked of the principal carer of someone with such an injury, not just as a support but as an interpreter, able to stand between their loved one and the world, explaining and excusing, protecting and encouraging. After months in this role, a close friend turned to Allan after a dinner in which he'd been doing all these things for Sheena and more, and asked him, 'What about you? Who is looking after you?' It was the first time since the accident that anyone had shown concern for his own well-being, and his reaction was to break down in sobs.

In 2019, I chaired a discussion between Sheena McDonald, Allan Little and Gail Robinson at the Edinburgh International Book Festival, exploring the challenges of recovery for patients, clinicians and carers. Gail spoke of how much Sheena's remarkable and enduring recovery was built on the solid foundation of Allan's support. For Allan, what ultimately helped was giving up on the idea that his life might return to the way it was before:

> It's a journey that changes the trajectory of your life, your priorities, your values, your hopes and ambitions, your sense of who you are in the world, and your relationship with those around you ... You are entering a new and unknown country, with an unfamiliar language and no map.

In a book on rehabilitation from brain injury the neuropsychologists Muriel Lezak and Thomas Kay suggest that 'the continual expectation of recovery can lead clients and families into denial, frustration and disappointment, and even worse, extremely unrealistic expectations and planning ... we prefer to speak in terms of hope for as much improvement as possible, to build in realistic expectations from the beginning'. It's a sobering thought, but recovery takes many forms. Allan's words on accepting that he and his partner's lives

had changed irrevocably brought to my mind Denise Riley's memoir of living with grief: *Time Lived, Without Its Flow*:

> your task now is to inhabit the only place left to you – the present instant – with equanimity, and in as much good heart as you can contrive.

12

TREATMENTS

There are few near-magical treatments in medicine, but 'convalescent plasma' can seem like one of them. This is the clear fluid extracted from blood that has been donated by someone who has suffered an illness and then recovered. Because the donor has been through the ordeal of a particular infectious disease, their blood is replete with antibodies that can fight that same disease in someone more vulnerable. Convalescent plasma isn't perfect as a treatment by any means, but by generating an immune response where none existed before it offers one of the best means we have of fighting an illness that our immune systems couldn't otherwise defeat.

One of the best defences against bacteria and viruses is prevention – having the strength and health to fight off infection. Convalescent plasma borrows the health and strength of one person and puts it in the service of another. In the early months of 2020, as the SARS-CoV2 pandemic spread around the globe, studies that tested different treatments for severe Covid-19 pneumonia used convalescent plasma as a gold standard treatment. The disease was so new that there were simply no other standards by which to compare.

This mode of protection is similar to the way in which nature works to safeguard newborn babies who, having grown in the pristine environment of the womb, would be utterly vulnerable to bacteria and viruses after birth without having received maternal antibodies that cross the placenta. Those antibodies prepare the baby to confront infection even before birth, and don't stop after delivery but switch to being carried over within breast milk instead. As long as breast-feeding contin-ues, the mother's body sends over antibodies against the viruses circulating in the community. From the outside it looks like a perfect cure.

But one of several problems with convalescent plasma is that antibodies are fickle things, fragile and prone to disintegration, and require frequent topping up. The plasma is also expensive to prepare, and from the perspective of the body, constitutes foreign material. A better (preventative) solution still is to have an effective vaccine, because vaccination teaches the body to create its own antibodies without risking the illness itself. But aside from a few exceptions (for example rabies), vaccination is of little use in the short term. It has to be embarked upon *before* the illness has begun. Throughout 2021 I saw the effectiveness of the Covid vaccine programme as month by month the progressively younger cohorts of the city were vaccinated, and hospital admission rates tumbled as a consequence.

Just as antibodies work better if our bodies create them themselves, the same can be said for the treatment of anaemia. When I was starting out in medicine we used to order a blood transfusion for anyone whose haemoglobin fell below about two-thirds of the normal level. But what we didn't know then is that funnelling someone else's blood into your veins might make the numbers on the lab tests look better – the haemoglobin figures always improved – but that the new blood didn't work properly. It was too old, stunned, somehow, by its time in the fridge, and foreign to the recipient. More recently it's been shown that it's better to let someone recover slowly from anaemia, building up their own blood through rest and good nutrition, than it is to pour in a couple of pints of someone else's. Sometimes, slow recoveries are the most effective kind.

A century ago doctors prescribed 'tonics' of all kinds to help with convalescence, and it's not easy now to figure out how much of the effectiveness of these medicines was down to the placebo effect. They usually contained iron, a bit of caffeine, and some vitamins. 'Easton's syrup', available as a liquid or in tablet form, had added quinine and strychnine, and was deemed so effective that polar explorers carried doses of it all the way to the South Pole and back. Lily the Pink's 'Vegetable Compound', which first became available in the 1870s, was called 'the greatest remedy in the world'. The famous powders of Thomas Beecham started out as tonic medicines. Every week or two I'm approached by a patient who wants me to prescribe a 'tonic' of one sort or another, reminding me that though scientific medicine has largely given up on ancient ideas of diet and nutriment as pivotal in recovery from illness, most of my patients haven't. When I was more inexperienced as a doctor I'd try to explain that I didn't hold much faith in tonics. But given that so many of my patients clearly did hold that faith, these days I'm more likely to take advantage of their ideas and print off a diet sheet. It's the least that some patients expect, and expectations are powerful remedies.

The idea that therapies must be something that you swallow or inject – that they should be pills, or syrups, or infusions – is wrong. For someone with Parkinson's disease, joining a dance club could be as effective as any medication they might take; someone with emphysema might be best advised to join a choir. Ballet and yoga improve strength and balance, and reduce the risk of falls, and I've known a walking or gardening club revolutionise someone's mental health, fitness and confidence. These kinds of recommendations are known as 'social prescribing' when they're given by doctors. But to join a group when you're lonely, or get active when you're sedentary, is simply common sense, and follows the old idea of health as a balance between extremes, not an extreme in itself.

For a gambling addict I knew, the most effective therapy was referral to a debt counsellor. For a woman struggling against drug dependency, starving herself to feed her habit, it was referral to a food bank. Having enough food in the cupboard gave her the peace of mind to be able to address her addiction. For a fit, newly retired and newly widowed man I knew, it was a volunteer agency that helped him the most.

For someone escaping an abusive marriage with her three children it was a phone call to the local branch of Women's Aid. For an immigrant family living in a damp, cramped slum it was a letter to the housing department.

It can be frustrating, as a doctor, to be faced with problems that have no medical solutions, and the expectation in wider society that therapies such as these *need* a doctor's referral can be equally frustrating. A recent UK government suggestion that doctors be given responsibility to prescribe vegetables is a case in point. There are those who, instead of addressing the social and economic causes of poor diet, prefer to rebrand poverty as a medical problem, and so pass it to health services to deal with. There's clearly nothing in particular about medical training that prepares a clinician for recommending clubs, better housing or food banks – 'treatments' that should be open to all. We shouldn't have to turn to doctors for the cure of problems that are social and political in nature, and it's often my impression that we already ask more of the health services than they are capable of providing. But for medicine to achieve its broadest goals it must embrace the broadest understanding of the roots of illness, whatever and wherever they are.

Hippocrates wrote that illness was influenced by the movement of the sun, qualities of the soil, and the prevailing winds, and in a sense he was right. We know now that there are deaths from air pollution, from nutritional deficiencies and toxins in soils, and that vitamin D from the sun influences our body's defences against illness (something seen most strikingly with Covid-19, when a correlation was uncovered between low vitamin D and extreme reactions to the illness). The justifiable fear of skin cancer has led pale-skinned people to shun sunshine, but for some that avoidance has become so extreme that their bones have weakened and their immune systems have suffered as a consequence.

And though therapies in their broadest sense might include a convalescent's blood, a mother's milk, drugs and tonics, singing and gardening, sun and wind, food banks and yoga,

there's another therapy that I occasionally recommend that can prove more effective than
any other.

The psychotherapist Carl Rogers pioneered
the idea that what any patient in emotional
and psychological distress needs is 'uncondi-
tional positive regard'. A few rare humans do
emanate this magnificent generosity of spirit
and speak with kindness and open compassion
to everyone, no matter how they might be
considered to have brought their sufferings on
themselves. But there's a shortcut, with a side
effect of promoting exercise, distraction from
your concerns, and constant companionship.
Get a pet.

13

THE (OCCASIONAL) ADVANTAGES OF ILLNESS

Some years ago now I looked after two men, both middle-aged, who a few weeks apart both suffered a cardiac arrest and collapsed, ostensibly dead, but who were successfully resuscitated with electric shocks. Both were then fitted with portable electronic defibrillators that were implanted beneath the skin of their left collarbones and wired directly into the heart. The defibrillators were about the shape and size of a matchbox or a Zippo lighter, and were clearly visible bulging under the skin. If either man was again to collapse with an erratic heartbeat, the portable defibrillator would sense the change and shock the heart back into a healthy rhythm.

For one of the men, his intimate experience of the proximity of death, the fragility of life and his new reliance on the implanted defibrillator was utterly traumatic. He began to suffer panic attacks and fiddled ceaselessly with the swelling beneath his collarbone. He couldn't find a way to stop fretting that it might fail. At the time of his cardiac arrest he had been working as an administrator, but he found himself unable to go on working. He was afraid to be alone, and his nights became a torment of insomnia.

For the other man, the almost identical experience of collapse and then resurrection became an epiphany of gratitude. His new life was a gift, he said, for by rights he should now be dead, and all the tedious, niggling irritations that once troubled him seemed to dissolve. It was enough to be able to breathe this air, walk on this earth, see his grandchildren. He had always lived modestly, but now began to enjoy sumptuous meals, fine wine, and booked holidays to places he would never before have considered visiting.

He had died, but then he lived again, and that new life into which he was born seemed one of richness, tenderness and gratitude.

That story reminded me of another reaction to near-death experience, one recounted by the novelist Maggie O'Farrell, who as a child almost died of encephalitis, an infection of the brain. Meningitis affects the brain's wrappings – the 'meninges' – but encephalitis affects the brain's cells themselves, and can be accordingly devastating in its effects. For O'Farrell it wasn't gratitude that became the strongest emotion of the many provoked by her illness, but the thrill of risk:

Nearly losing my life at the age of eight made me sanguine – perhaps to a fault – about death. I knew it would happen, at some point, and the idea didn't scare me; its proximity felt instead almost familiar. The knowledge that I was lucky to be alive, that it could so easily have been otherwise, skewed my thinking. I viewed my continuing life as an extra, a bonus, a boon: I could do with it what I wanted. And not only had I tricked death but I had escaped a fate of incapacity. What else was I going to do with my independence, my ambulatory state, except exploit it for all that it was worth?

The clinical psychologist Lisl Marburg Goodman proposed that for some of her patients illness brought an awareness of mortality that could, like my second patient with his defibrillator, help to cherish the moment. In her book *Death and the Creative Life* Marburg Goodman advised that, instead of calculating our age from birth, we calculate the year at which we might reasonably expect to die, and count backwards to the years we have left: 'in this way we would keep life, and death, always in front of us.'

It's not easy to live in the glaring knowledge of life's brevity, whatever gifts that knowledge might grant, and it changes people profoundly. In a long essay titled 'Living in the Present', the

philosopher Havi Carel wrote of the way reconciliation with a rare and life-threatening lung
condition had occasioned a transformation of
her perspective on time:

> Time did change for me. I began to take
> it much more seriously. I began to make a
> point of enjoying things thoroughly: mem-
> orizing sensations, views, moments. Partly
> in preparation for days to come in which I
> may not be able to leave the house or my
> bed, but also in order to feel that I have
> taken the time to really sense, really expe-
> rience pleasurable things. I wanted to feel
> that I am living life to the full in the present.
> That I *am* now.

Life, for Carel, is like a river, and to live with a
severe chronic illness is to see that river become
'a tempestuous series of rapids'. Each set of
rapids is a crisis in the evolution of illness,
but their very turmoil means that calm inter-
ludes become all the more precious. The list
of things that might go wrong with our bodies

is terrifying but that list is a manifestation of a truth that is real for all of us: life can be taken away at any moment. At one level, convalescence has something in common with dying in that it forces us to engage with our limitations, the fragile nature of our existence. Why not, then, live fully while we can?

Carel quotes Nietzsche, for whom convalescence's meaning of 'strength returning' was a joyous experience: 'It was as if I discovered life anew, myself included; I tasted all the good things, even the small ones, as no other could easily taste them.' Elsewhere, Nietzsche wrote of how the predominant emotion of recovery was a sense of thanks: 'Gratitude pours forth continually, as if the unexpected had just happened – the gratitude of a convalescent – for convalescence was unexpected.'

I remember a young woman I encountered early in my GP training who had been struck by a bus while out cycling, and whose recovery took more than a year of surgical operations, her bones repeatedly re-broken and reset. The experience was almost unbearable, but at the same time it occasioned the discovery of an inner strength that she didn't know she possessed. Her priorities shifted, and she became determined to live on with a ferocity and intensity that, without the injuries, she never would have known. We make our own realities, as I saw with the two men who suffered identical, traumatic near-death experiences, were resurrected by defibrillators, but who interpreted those experiences in diametrically opposed ways.

Anatole Broyard's book about his prostate cancer, *Intoxicated by My Illness*, is one of the most thoughtful and meditative books on reconciliation to illness that I know of. 'As I look ahead, I feel like a man who has awakened from a long afternoon nap to find the evening stretched out before me,' he wrote. Rather than finding his new awareness of his mortality depressing, the brevity of the time he might have left to live charged his days with grandeur and beauty. 'I see the balance of my life as a beautiful paisley shawl thrown over a grand piano.' Even the news of his cancer was welcomed in its way; it was 'like an immense electric shock. I felt galvanized. I was a new person. All my old trivial selves fell away, and I was reduced to essence.'

If we can take any gifts or wisdom from the experience of illness, surely it's this: to deepen our appreciation of health, and make us appreciate what we have in the knowledge that it can so easily be taken away.

CONCLUSIONS

The founding constitution of the World Health Organization gives its stated definition of health as 'a state of complete physical, mental and social well-being and not merely the absence of disease and infirmity'. If we take that as the aim of recovery, none of us have any chance at all. My own view of health is less demanding and I hope might be more in reach. 'Health' means 'wholeness' but there are many ways of remaking our selves towards that state, and of rebuilding elements of our lives after illness. Rather than a destination in and of itself, recovery is better thought of as something dynamic, just like life – a direction of travel that we can be guided towards. Anyone whose life is moving in the direction of more dignity, understanding, and in accord with their wishes, is in some sense on a journey of recovery.

Professor Christopher Ward, a clinician and academic specialist in rehabilitation medicine, asks his patients with chronic illness what they would have missed of their lives if they had never become ill. In his book *Between Sickness and Health* he explains that the answers he has received over the years have been diverse: from couples who felt that their relationship had deepened, to individuals who had been exposed to 'previously unimagined possibilities'. One woman described the strength she had gathered through living with chronic fatigue, and how it had made her less evasive as a person – more able to confront the difficulties in her life. For Ward, it is tyrannous to assume that positivity can overcome all obstacles, and he reminds his readers that much of what constitutes illness consists of things we cannot change. His first step with a new patient is always to acknowledge the suffering they have experienced and continue to experience, and to then redefine the goals of treatment not necessarily as 'rehabilitation' but as 'possibilitation': the opportunity of each person to fulfil their potential, to be the best *possible* version of themselves. Considering how to get to a unique version of wholeness appropriate for each of us, he invokes Reinhold Niebuhr's famous serenity prayer:

grant me the serenity to accept the things I
  cannot change,
the courage to change the things I can,
    and the wisdom to know the difference.

No one can be talked out of chronic physical, mental or emotional pain, but it's within our power to change our expectations of recovery, and with that, I've seen people in the most trying of situations find ways to keep hope alive. Though we often can't overcome illness, we can find ways to improve our circumstances, and live with it in a sort of negotiated peace.

Even with the advances of twenty-first-century

tech-medicine, surgery, DNA profiling and gene therapy, the list of illnesses that can be definitively cured is surprisingly short. But for all that Western medicine frequently disappoints, it remains a powerful approach to the body and its failings, and for that reason has been adopted in some form or another almost everywhere in the world. Even its ability to define and name our illnesses can offer consolation – I've seen many patients reassured by that act of naming, comforted by the knowledge that what afflicts them has an existence separate from themselves. The naming of an illness offers access to a community of others who have found ways of living with the same difficulties, and that itself can be a source of hope.

But there's a paradox at work: categorising an illness can offer a false sense of definition, locking us into an expectation that becomes self-fulfilling. The reality of both mind and body is one of dynamism and change; any vision of human life that is static at heart is an illusion. When a patient tells me 'I've *got* that depression' I know that part of my job will be to guide that patient back towards a more fluid understanding of mood, and a more hopeful perspective on their mental state. I've found that the most helpful approach is not to think of illness categories as concrete, immutable destinies but as stories of the mind and the body. Within limits, stories can be rewritten.

No one is getting any younger, and all of us would do well to remember that health can never be a final destination, but a balance between extremes, different for everyone, and whether we reach it or not depends on our goals and priorities as much as it depends on anatomy and physiology. There is no one-size-fits-all in medicine, and though in these pages I've tried to set out a few ideas about recovery and convalescence, I'm conscious that it's possible to touch on only a few of them. I hope that these reflections, experiences and principles might prove helpful to some. Though they may not offer an escape route out of the landscape of illness, they might at least help to orientate the map.

So give time, space and respect to convalescence if you can. It's an act that we need
to engage in, giving of ourselves; a work of
effort and endurance, and to a certain extent
of grace. Charge your environment with as
much as you're able of space, light, cleanliness,
greenery, quiet. Remember that healing isn't a
game of snakes and ladders: with each movement towards and away from health we have
more than dice to guide us, and with every
cycle of boom and bust we gather experience
that will help us, next time. Learn a new language of the body and listen to it with care.
Get a sick note if you need one, but beware of
letting your horizons get too narrow, or your
confidence fall, because we are social beings
who need to act in the world, and work can
help us accomplish that. Everyone needs activity of one kind or another. Take a sabbatical if
you can, and don't worry too much over the
time it might take to recover: everyone's tempo
of recovery is different, and subject to different
pressures. Travel if you can, and if you can't,
travel vicariously through the stories of others

or through books. Attend to your surroundings and your occupations and if they're making you sick, change them. Think about your diet, and whether it's a help or a hindrance to recovery. Health is a balance: rest, but not too much; get active, but not too much. Find a clinician you trust. Don't expect all doctors and nurses to be the same: it's good that they're all different – they're fallible individuals, and are usually trying their best. Remember the needs and the frustrations of carers and those around you. Be your own best physician: drugs are the least of healing, and there are many kinds of therapies – singing, walking, eating, dancing, or sitting in the sunshine with a beloved pet on your lap. And for all its irritations and frustrations, its agonies and humiliations, illness is a part of life that may teach something of value, even if that thing is only to cherish health when we have it, or see it in others. Doctors and nurses are more like gardeners than mechanics, and healing happens thanks to the same force that greens the trees in spring and pushes bulbs up through the earth. Be kind to yourself. Take care over

who you listen to, because ideas and expectations are as powerful as drugs and poisons.
Human beings understand the world through
stories: not all will have a happy ending, but
each of us has a hand in writing part of our
own.

THANKS

Abraham Verghese, Allan Little, Andrew Franklin, Andy Elder, Atul Gawande, Brian Dean, Calum Morrison, Cecily Gayford, Claudia Galante, Colin Speight, David McNeish, Esa Aldegheri, Fiona Wright, Flora Willis, Francesca Barrie, Gail Robinson, Geraldine Fraser, Hannah Ross, Iona Heath, Ishbel White, Iwona Stolarek, Janis Blair, Jenna Pemberton, Jenny Brown, Jim Gallagher, Jinty Francis, John Goodall, John Murphy, Jon Stone, Jude Henderson, Julie Craig, Kate Edgar, Lindsey McDonald, Malcolm Fraser, Michael Stein, Mike Ferguson, Mimi Cogliano, Nicola Gray, Pearl Ferguson, Peter Dorward, Peter Dyer, Rebecca Sutherland, Sandy Reid, Sharon Lawson, Sheena McDonald, Susanne Hillen, Suzanne O'Sullivan, Valentina Zanca.

And with much gratitude to: Havi Carel, for permitting me to quote from *Illness* (Routledge, 2013); Jay Griffiths, for permitting me to quote from *Tristimania* (Hamish Hamilton, 2016); John Launer, for permitting me to quote from *How Not to Be a Doctor* (Duckworth, 2018); Maggie O'Farrell, for permitting me to quote from 'Cerebellum' in *I Am I Am I Am* (Tinder Press, 2018); Victoria Sweet, for permitting me to quote from *God's Hotel* (Riverhead, 2012); and Christopher Ward, for permitting me to quote from *Between Sickness and Health* (Routledge, 2020).

NOTES ON SOURCES

2: Hospitals and Recovery

12 'Between 1800 and 1914 the ...' and 'Between 1860 and 1980 the UK ...' Roy Porter, *The Greatest Benefit to Mankind* (London: Fontana, 1999).

13 'signify the proper use ...' Florence Nightingale, *Notes on Nursing: What it is, and What it is Not* (London: Harrison, 1860).

13 'a recommendation that has been ...' R. S. Ulrich, 'View through a window may influence recovery from surgery', *Science* 224 (1984), 420–21.

13 'I am a kind of General ...', from *The Greatest Benefit to Mankind*.

15 'Average lifespans around the world ...' Ian Goldin and Robert Muggah, *Terra Incognita: 100 Maps to Survive the Next 100 Years* (London: Century, 2020).

3: Snakes and Ladders

20   '... to be built up slowly after injury ...' See Galen, *De Exercitio Per Parvam Pilam* in John Redman Coxe, *The Writings of Hippocrates and Galen. Epitomised from the Original Latin translations* (Philadelphia: Lindsay & Blakiston, 1846).

21   NHS Lothian Covid Recovery Booklet, 2020, distributed as a PDF to GPs.

4: Permission to Recover

24   'work in partnership ...' General Medical Council, *Good Medical Practice* (London: GMC, 2013, updated November 2020).

24   'doctors make terrible referees ...' to 'over-claimed through "genuine error"' Adrian Massey, *Sick-Note Britain* (London: Hurst, 2019).

31   'enforced pursuit of an activity ...' P. B. Lieberman and J. S. Strauss, 'The recurrence of mania: environmental factors and medical treatment', *The American Journal of Psychiatry* 141 (1984), 77–80.

32   'Dealing with the links between poverty ...' Hellen Matthews and John Bain (eds), *Doctors Talking* (Edinburgh: Scottish Cultural Press, 1998).

33   'falling ill, and especially ...' Michael Balint, *The*

Doctor, His Patient & the Illness (London: Pitman, 1957).

35   'Modern methods of ...' Bertrand Russell, 'In Praise of Idleness', *Harper's Magazine*, October 1932.

37   'in the rhythm of life ...' Rabindranath Tagore, *Glorious Thoughts of Tagore* (Delhi: New Book Society of India, 1965).

37   'when one can feel that one's work ...' Oliver Sacks, 'Sabbath' in *Gratitude* (London: Knopf, 2015).

38   'The original sabbaticals were a ...' Theodore Zeldin, *An Intimate History of Humanity* (London: Vintage, 1994).

5: Travel

40   'very often the cure is effected ...' Cicero, *Tusculan Disputations IV*, trans. J. E. King (Cambridge, MA: Harvard University Press/ Loeb Classical Library 141, 1971), 35.

41   'Darwin noted that ...' Charles Darwin, *On the Origin of Species* (London: John Murray, 1859).

41   'And specially, from every shire's ...' Geoffrey Chaucer, Prologue, *The Canterbury Tales* (Harmondsworth: Penguin, 1963).

44   'as a holiday, and a refreshment ...' J. R. R. Tolkien, *Tree and Leaf* (London: HarperCollins, 1988).

6: The Architecture of Recovery

48 'Mr David Ainslie of Costerton ...' Lothian
    Health Archive: https://www.lhsa.lib.ed.ac.uk/
    exhibits/hosp_hist/astley_ainslie.htm, accessed
    September 2021.

7: The Rest Cure

51 '[you] order rest in bed ...' Virginia Woolf, *Mrs
    Dalloway* (Oxford: Oxford University Press,
    2000).

53 'Millions of dead molecules are ...' Silas Weir
    Mitchell, 'Convalescence' in *Doctor and Patient*,
    (Philadelphia: Lippincott, 1901).

55 'over-stressed business executives of both ...'
    Anne Stiles, 'Go rest, young man', *Journal of the
    American Psychological Association* 43 (2012), 32.

8: Back to Nature

60 'What then was life? ...' Thomas Mann, *The
    Magic Mountain*, trans. H.T. Lowe-Porter
    (London: Vintage, 1999).

61 'In her book *God's Hotel* ...' Victoria Sweet, *God's
    Hotel* (New York: Riverhead, 2012).

63 'Today all that we have left ...', from *God's Hotel*.

9: The Ideal Doctor

65 'It is much more important ...' William Osler,

in *The Quotable Osler* (Philadelphia: American College of Physicians, 2008).

66 'I've got three problems ...' John Launer, *How Not to Be a Doctor* (London: Duckworth, 2018).

68 'spontaneity and intuitive understanding ...' Donald Winnicott, 'Skin Changes in Relation to Emotional Disorder' (1938) in *The Collected Works of D. W. Winnicott* Volume 8 (Oxford: Oxford University Press, 2017).

69 'The confidence (or lack of) which a doctor ...' Jay Griffiths, *Tristimania* (London: Hamish Hamilton, 2016).

72 'St Luke was a doctor ...' Anatole Broyard, *Intoxicated by My Illness* (New York: Ballantine, 1992).

74 'Doctor-as-guide is an ancient idea ...' For more on St Basil see Abraham Nussbaum, *The Finest Traditions of My Calling* (New Haven: Yale University Press, 2016).

10: Writing Your Own Story

77 'it was Queequeg's conceit ...' Herman Melville, *Moby Dick* (New York: Harper, 1851).

78 Re. colours of placebos: see for example A. J. M. de Craen et al., 'Effect of colour of drugs: systematic review of perceived effect of drugs and of their effectiveness', *BMJ* 313 (1996), 1624–6.

79   'specialising in what are now called …' Suzanne
     O'Sullivan, *It's All in Your Head* (London: Chatto
     & Windus, 2015).

81   'The Hmong suggested that …' Suzanne
     O'Sullivan, *The Sleeping Beauties* (London:
     Picador, 2021).

11: On Carers

86   'Through the Covid pandemic it has been
     estimated …' *Unseen and Undervalued – Carers UK
     Report*, November 2020.

88   'In the book they wrote together …' Sheena
     McDonald, Allan Little and Gail Robinson,
     Rebuilding Life after Brain Injury (Abingdon:
     Routledge, 2019).

90   'the continual expectation …' Thomas Kay and
     Muriel Lezak, chapter 2, 'The nature of head
     injury', in D. W. Corthell (ed.), *Traumatic Brain
     Injury and Vocational Rehabilitation* (Menomonie:
     University of Wisconsin, 1990).

91   'your task now is …' Denise Riley, *Time Lived,
     Without Its Flow* (London: Picador, 2019).

13: The (occasional) Advantages of Illness

103 'Nearly losing my life …' Maggie O'Farrell, from
     'Cerebellum' in *I Am I Am I Am* (London: Tinder
     Press, 2018).

104 'in this way we would keep …' Lisl Marburg
Goodman, *Death and the Creative Life*
(Harmondsworth: Penguin, 1983).

105 'Time did change for me …' Havi Carel, *Illness*
(Abingdon: Routledge, 2013).

106 'It was as if I discovered …' Friedrich
Nietzsche, *Ecce Homo*, trans. R. J. Hollingdale
(Harmondsworth: Penguin, 1992).

106 'Gratitude pours forth …' Friedrich Nietzsche,
The Gay Science, trans. W. A. Kaufmann (London:
Vintage, 1974).

107 'As I look ahead …' to 'reduced to essence'
Anatole Broyard, *Intoxicated by My Illness* (New
York: Ballantine, 1992).

Conclusions

110 'previously unimagined possibilities' Christopher
Ward, *Between Sickness and Health* (Abingdon:
Routledge, 2020).

111 'grant me the serenity …' Reinhold Niebuhr,
'The Serenity Prayer', for which see, for
example, Elisabeth Sifton, *The Serenity Prayer:
Faith and Politics in Times of Peace and War* (New
York: W. W. Norton, 2005).

ABOUT THE AUTHOR

A doctor who views medicine as the 'alliance of science and kindness', Gavin Francis has worked across four continents as a surgeon, emergency physician, medical officer with the British Antarctic Survey and latterly as a GP. He is the author of the *Sunday Times* bestseller *Adventures in Human Being, Shapeshifters* and *Intensive Care*, an account of the Covid-19 pandemic. He also writes for the *Guardian*, *The Times*, the *London Review of Books* and *Granta*.

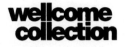

WELLCOME COLLECTION publishes thought-provoking books exploring health and human experience, in partnership with leading independent publisher Profile Books.

WELLCOME COLLECTION is a free museum and library that aims to challenge how we think and feel about health by connecting science, medicine, life and art, through exhibitions, collections, live programming, and more. It is part of Wellcome, a global charitable foundation that supports science to solve urgent health challenges, with a focus on mental health, infectious diseases and climate.

wellcomecollection.org